Author

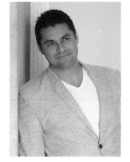

As a medical professional and healer
I believe in "an apple a day keeps the
doctor away" approach. Prevention
is better than cure. With the exploding
and evolving field of probiotics and
focus on the association between
gut bacteria and various diseases,
I think the next decade will be
revolutionary.

> – Rajiv K. Sharma MD
> *Gastroenterologist*

author

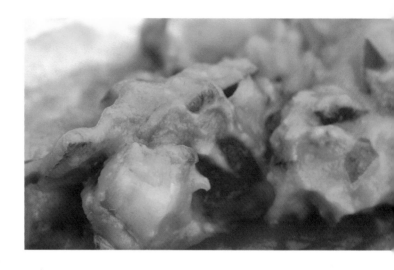

Pursuit of Gut Happiness

A guide for using probiotics
to achieve optimal health

RAJIV K. SHARMA MD
Board Certified Gastroenterologist
Wellness Physician
Self-Proclaimed Gastronomist

1st Edition

LIMITATION OF LIABILITY STATEMENT

Probiotics are considered dietary supplements; thus, they are not covered by medical insurance and their production is not regulated by the Food and Drug Administration. As such, product quality, purity and viability have been reported to be variable. Please keep your allergies, food and flavor preferences and health problems in mind before trying any probiotics, fermented foods and probiotic recipes, including but not limited to the ones mentioned in this book and associated websites/social media.

Although every effort has been made to provide complete and accurate information, Rajiv Sharma MD, RAAMS Consulting LLC its affiliates, associates & subsidiaries make no warranties, express or implied, or representations as to the accuracy of content in this book(s), on the associated website(s) or social media networks. Rajiv Sharma MD, RAAMS Consulting LLC and its affiliates, associates & subsidiaries assume no liability or responsibility for any errors or omissions in the information contained in this book(s), the website(s) or its social networks and the operation of the website or its social media networks.

This book(s), the associated website(s) and social media networks contain general information about medical conditions and treatments. The information is not advice, and should not be treated as such. The contents of this work (publications, websites, social media networks, blogs) are intended to promote general understanding, discussion and awareness ONLY and should not be perceived or relied upon as authoritative recommendation or promotion of a specific diagnostic or treatment approach by physicians for any patients or self treatment by the readers. Readers need to be aware that the field of science is constantly and rapidly evolving due to the influx of new research, publications, governmental regulations and constant flow of information relating to the use of medicines, medical equipment, health foods, health supplements, medical foods and medical devices. Please refer to the information provided in the package insert on the manufacturer's website so you can carefully follow and understand the instructions or indications for usage such as dose, frequency, precautions, warnings, storing instructions and other risk factors. PREGNANT and lactating persons need to talk to their health care provider before following any information provided in this book(s), on the associated website(s), blogs or social media networks. PLEASE CONSULT A SPECIALIST WHEN YOU NEED MORE INFORMATION. DO NOT ASSUME ANY INFORMATION OR INSTRUCTION.

By using this book(s), RAAMS Consulting LLC's websites, blogs or its social media networks, you assume all risks associated with the use of the above sources including any risk of your computer, software or data being damaged by a virus, software or any other files that might be transmitted or activated via the use of the above mentioned book(s), website(s), links, blogs and/or social media networks.

Rajiv Sharma MD, RAAMS Consulting LLC and its affiliates, associates & subsidiaries expressly disclaim any and all liability for any special, incidental or consequential damages, including without limitation, medical & health related problems, lost revenues or lost profits resulting from the use or misuse of the information contained in the book(s), publications, website(s) or its social networks.

LIMITATION OF WARRANTIES

The medical information on this website is provided "as is" without any representations or warranties, express or implied. Rajiv Sharma MD, RAAMS Consulting LLC and its affiliates, associates & subsidiaries make no representations, guarantees or warranties in relation to the medical and non-medical information in this book(s), publications, associated websites and social media sites.

Without prejudice to the generality of the foregoing paragraph, Rajiv Sharma MD, RAAMS Consulting LLC and its affiliates, associates & subsidiaries warrant that:

1. The medical information on this website will be constantly available, or available at all; or
2. The medical information on this website is complete, true, accurate, up-to-date or non-misleading.

PROFESSIONAL ASSISTANCE

You must NOT rely on the information in this book(s), publications, blogs, associated website(s) and social media sites as an alternative to medical advice from your doctor or other professional healthcare provider. If you have any specific questions about any medical matter you should consult your doctor or other professional healthcare provider. Pregnant women, those within child bearing age and lactating persons need to exercise extreme caution and common sense when interpreting the above information.

If you think you may be suffering from any medical condition you should seek medical attention immediately. You should never delay seeking medical advice, disregard medical advice or discontinue medical treatment because of information in this book(s), publications, blogs, associated website(s) and social media sites.

LIABILITY

Nothing in this medical disclaimer will limit any of our liabilities in any way that is not permitted under applicable law, or exclude any of our liabilities that may not be excluded under applicable law.

INDEMNIFICATION

You agree to defend, indemnify and hold Rajiv Sharma MD, RAAMS Consulting LLC

Please direct all inquiries to:
RAAMS CONSULTING LLC
www.rajivksharmamd.com
phone: 312-880-7775

An introduction to the world of probiotics.

This book is your first step toward diving deep into the ocean of information about probiotics, so to speak "baby steps." I don't call this "the bible," but after reading this book, I want you to feel comfortable, to be able to understand the word probiotic, and carry on a two-minute conversation with Grandpa Moses or Aunt Sally.

– RAJIV K. SHARMA MD

Table of Contents

contents

Recipes

Liquids

Solids

Chapter 1

PROBIOTICS: "FOR LIFE"

SHALL I TAKE A PROBIOTIC? I HEARD IT HELPS MAINTAIN GOOD HEALTH. "My mother takes one, I just cannot think of the name!" "My sister's health care provider said to take one daily. I just don't know which one to take." I get asked this question all the time, not just by patients but also by friends and co-workers.

There is almost a fanaticism about probiotics. Commercial firms have jumped headfirst into this multi-billion dollar market. Heck, why not? Achieving optimal health and fitness is everyone's new year resolution. Health expense is the biggest concern of any family or individual. Our trillion dollar health care industry is driven by fear of ill health and treatment of ill health. The market has exploded with a gazillion probiotics. Everyone and their grandmother is trying to make their own probiotic.

When I Googled "probiotics for health," the search brought back about 24,400,000 results in 0.36 seconds. Probiotics are sold in many forms: pills, fermented milks (*animal based: cow, buffalo, camel, goat, donkey and vegetable based: soy, coconut, rice, wheat, pea, etc.*), powders, yogurts and kefir. Many companies are trying to use advanced biotechnology to produce high quality probiotic fortified infant formulas. Probiotics help to reduce colic and functional gastrointestinal disorders in infants. To qualify as probiotic, the food product needs to have active cultures. Even though the common yogurt has healthy lactobacilli bacteria, it does not qualify as probiotic until it has "active cultures." So, always look at the label carefully.

- http://www.nutraingredients.com/Industry/Italians-target-infants-with-donkey-milk-probiotics
- http://www.nutraingredients.com/Industry/Irish-firm-offers-cheaper-heat-resistant-probiotics-for-infant-formula

WHAT IS A PROBIOTIC?

SO WHAT IS A PROBIOTIC? Probiotics are defined by the World Health Organization as "live micro-organisms that can provide benefits to human health when administered in adequate amounts, which confer a beneficial health effect on the host" (*WHO/2001*). Probiotics are mainly bacteria, but can be yeast (*fungus*).

Gastric acid is the body's defense and kills the bacteria and fungi, so this is another "ocean of death" the probiotics need to swim through to survive and populate the rest of the gastrointestinal tract.

To qualify as a probiotic, the micro-organisms should be hardy and demonstrate:

- Resistance to gastric acidity
- Bile acid resistance (*bile acids help in digestion and absorption of food nutrients*)
- Attachment to mucus and/or human epithelial cells and cell lines
- Antimicrobial activity against potentially pathogenic bacteria
- Ability to reduce pathogen adhesion to surfaces
- Bile salt hydrolase activity (*break down bile salts to simpler substrates*)
- Resistance to spermicides (*applicable to probiotics for vaginal use*)

There is a unique nomenclature for probiotics. It is necessary to know the genus and species (*classification criteria*) of the probiotic strain. The current state of evidence suggests that probiotic effects are strain specific.

Strain identity is important to link a strain to a specific health effect as well as to enable accurate surveillance and epidemiological studies. Historically, *Lactobacilli (has multiple species)* and *Bifidobacteria (has multiple species)* associated with food have been considered to be safe *(Adams & Marteau, 1995)*. Their occurrence as normal commensals of the mammalian flora and their established safe use in a diversity of foods and supplement products worldwide supports this conclusion.

I will try to answer the following questions in this book. I will not go into endless details. My goal is to keep it fun and simple to maintain your interest. For any unanswered questions you can visit my website www.rajivksharmamd.com, email us at raamsconsultingllc@gmail.com, or speak with your physician.

1. Which probiotic should I take?
2. Which probiotic is better for my condition?
3. Which probiotic is the best?
4. Is it safe to take probiotics?
5. How long should I take it?
6. There are so many of these in the market, I am confused!
7. Is it safe? Is it FDA approved?

Since there is a gray zone when it comes to probiotics compared to simple healthy bacteria such as the *Lactobacilli* found in yogurt, the WHO/FAO Working Group *(2001)* recommends that the following information be described on the label of probiotic product(s):

1. Genus, species and strain designation. Strain designation should not mislead consumers about the functionality of the strain
2. Minimum viable numbers of each probiotic strain at the end of the shelf life

3. The suggested serving size must deliver the effective dose of probiotics related to the health claim

4. Health claim(s)

5. Proper storage conditions

6. Corporate contact details for consumer information

Probiotics are considered dietary supplements, thus they are routinely not covered by medical insurance and their production is not regulated by the Food and Drug Administration. As such, product quality, purity and viability have been reported to be variable.

- http://www.who.int/foodsafety/publications/fs_management/en/probiotics.pdf?ua=1

Quoted from: Joint FAO/WHO Expert Consultation on Evaluation of Health and Nutritional Properties of Probiotics in Food Including Powder Milk with Live Lactic Acid Bacteria, October 2001

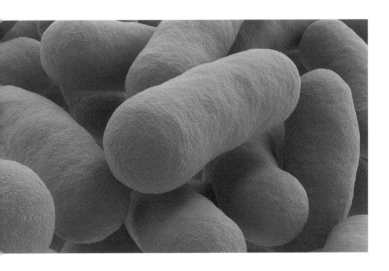

Chapter 2

GUT IS AN ECOSYSTEM:
Gut and Bacteria "Talk to Each Other"

PER WEBSTER'S DICTIONARY, "ECOSYSTEM" IS DEFINED AS "THE COMPLEX OF A COMMUNITY OF ORGANISMS AND ITS ENVIRONMENT FUNCTIONING AS AN ECOLOGICAL UNIT." Hence, the various life forms co-exist and interact. The human gut has more than 500 species of commensal *(natural inhabitant)* bacteria, plus yeast and viral species. Gut microbes can weigh up to 1 kilogram. These gut microbes interact with the immune system to a great extent.

The human gut has a lot of immune cells, even more than the bone marrow. The gut microbiome seems to have a role in inflammatory bowel diseases such as Crohn's disease and ulcerative colitis, bacterial vaginosis *(overgrowth of pathogenic bacteria in the vagina)*, asthma and allergies.

New research has also linked obesity and mood disorders to dysbiosis *(imbalance of gut bacteria)*. The gut bacteria help to maintain local defense by competing with pathogenic microbes, which are mostly bacteria but could also be fungi or viruses. The competition for nutrients and space, as well as secretion of certain bio-chemicals, inhibits the growth of these "invaders."

Gut bacteria produce SCFAs, or short chain fatty acids (*eg: butyric acid, propionic acid etc.*), which change the pH of the colon thereby inhibiting the growth of bad bacteria. The colonization of the gut by specific bacteria is dependent on interaction between the gut bacteria, host (*human cells*) and the gut immune system.

Major proteins in human blood are albumin and globulin. Globulins are proteins that play a role in immune defense mechanisms. IgA (*Immunoglobulin*) is a special type of globulin defense antibody that resides on the mucosa of the human intestine and other mucous membranes. It is one of the soldiers in body's "antibody" defense and guards the area where the mucosal linings interact with the outside environmental agents. There is ongoing extensive research to establish relation between gut bacteria and various diseases. Since the future of health care and medical treatment is DNA and genetic code driven, the next decade(s) will see more emphasis on deciphering the "Gut Microbiome Code" much akin to the "Da Vinci Code." The National Institute of Health (*NIH*) has initiated a "HMP": Human Microbiome Project (*sounds like a secret CIA project*), which will attempt to decode the DNA and genetic material of all the gut bacteria. This will help us use a more focused approach to tailor medical treatment. For example, instead of the whole probiotic we can identify the gene coding for a certain beneficial protein product, which could be collected, stored and distributed to achieve the desired effect. Its almost like drinking fruit juice without having to chew the entire fruit.

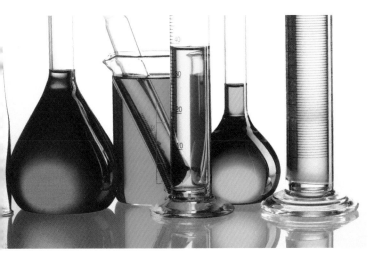

Chapter 3
WE NEED OUR GUT BACTERIA

GUT BACTERIA ARE THERE FOR A PURPOSE. THEY ARE NATURE'S GATEKEEPERS. Gut bacteria have a multitude of functions. They maintain local defense to ward off pathogenic or "bad bacteria" by competing for food and space as well as producing certain by-products that inhibit the growth of pathogens. They produce good vitamins such as vitamin K (*helps to make blood clotting factors*) and folic acid (*a type of B vitamin, typically found in green leafy vegetables*). They produce short chain fatty acids (SCFAs), which are a source of energy and have a role in suppressing inflammation. Gut micro-organisms are important for adequate development of the human immune system. The gut is an immune organ and almost 90% of human immune cells reside there. Just like the brain, the gut also has neurotransmitters, the special chemicals that relay nerve signals. The gut has more than 30 neurotransmitters, namely serotonin, acetylcholine, nitric oxide, Vasoactive Intestinal Peptide (*VIP*), Cholecystokinin (*CCK*), Tachykinins and Substance P, to name a few. Ninety percent of the body's neurotransmitter serotonin (*the happiness chemical*) is found in the gut. Serotonin plays a role in motility, peristalsis and pain sensitivity of the gut. In-depth discussion about these chemicals is beyond the scope of my message.

The gut microbes and their products have an impact on secretions of certain chemicals and hormones from the lining of the intestine, which in turn has an effect on healing of the gut lining in that region.

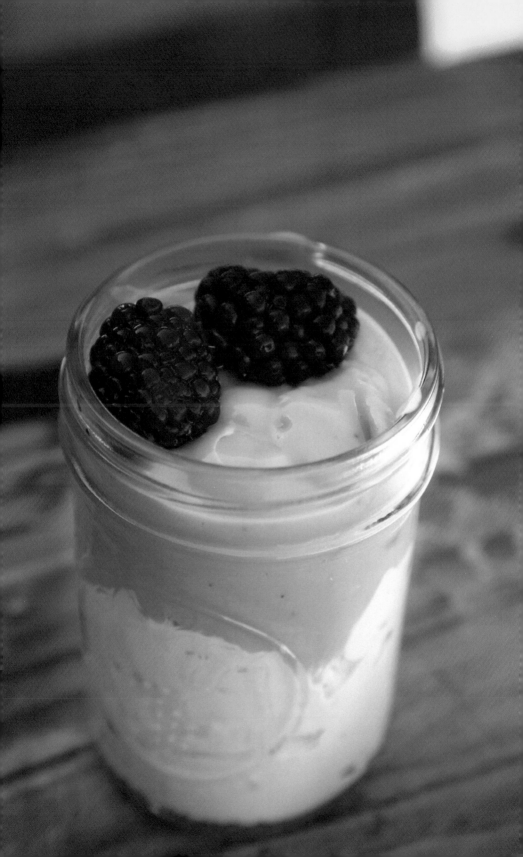

Chapter 4

METCHNIKOFF'S "SOUR MILK" FOR YOUTHFULNESS

NOBEL PRIZE WINNING, RUSSIAN BORN SCIENTIST ELIE METCHNIKOFF (*born 1845*) is considered the grandfather of the probiotics concept and its health benefits. He worked at the Pasteur Institute in France where he performed extensive research in the field of microbiology. He had observed that Bulgarian peasants enjoyed good health due to their consumption of fermented sour milk. He linked this to the "Bulgarian bacillus," which was discovered by a Bulgarian physician, Stamen Grigorov, who also demonstrated that healthy bacteria in yogurt help with digestion and improve the immune system.

Metchnikoff proposed the use of *Bulgarian bacillus* (*now known as Lactobacillus delbrueckii*) to treat colon afflictions. In 1904, he became the deputy director at the Pasteur Institute laboratory in Paris and worked extensively on phagocytosis (*phenomenon where immune cells engulf and destroy invading agents*) and inflammation. For this work, he was awarded the Nobel Prize for medicine in 1908.

At the same time as Elie Metchnikoff, Henry Tissier, a French pediatrician, observed that stools of children with diarrhea had a low number of bacteria characterized by a peculiar Y shaped morphology. These "bifid" bacteria were, on the contrary, abundant in healthy children (*Tissier, 1906*). He suggested that these bacteria could be administered to patients with diarrhea to help restore a healthy gut flora. *Escherichia coli* and *Bifidobacterium* have been used in the late 1880s and 1950s to treat various digestive track afflictions. Unfortunately at that time, the antibiotic era was just taking off so the probiotics concept was not taken very seriously.

In the early 1900s, Metchnikoff regularly drank a preparation of a pure "sour milk" made by using special lactic ferment or "culture," which he selected and cultivated himself. The scientific rationale for the health benefit of lactic acid bacteria was provided in his book, "The Prolongation of Life" published in 1907.

Elie Metchnikoff's life and work is beautifuly captured in his biography called "Life of Elie Metchnikoff, 1845-1916," by Olga Metchnikoff, a friend and colleague (*a translated from French to English version is available for free www.gutenberg.org*).

- ftp://ftp.fao.org/docrep/fao/009/a0512e/a0512e00.pdf

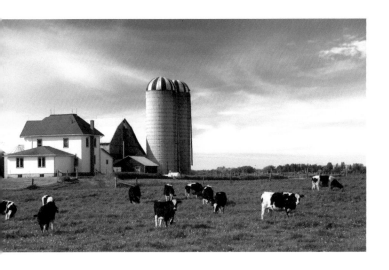

Chapter 5

SAFETY OF PROBIOTICS

IT IS NORMAL TO WONDER WHETHER TAKING "MICROBE SUPPLEMENT" IS SAFE. The great majority of probiotics are safe, especially in a normal healthy person. Studies suggest that probiotics usually have few side effects. However, the data on safety, particularly long-term safety, is limited, and the risk of serious side effects may be greater in people who have underlying health conditions where the immune system is compromised and cannot fight the invading pathogens:

1. Immunosuppressive disorders such as HIV
   (*HIV virus suppresses the immune system*)

2. Patients receiving chemotherapy
   (*chemotherapy shuts down the immune function*)

3. Patients on immune suppressing drugs
   for example: Remicade®, Humira®, Cimzia®, Methotrexate, Mercaptopurine, etc.)

4. Patients with congenital or genetic immunosuppressive disorders

5. Patients sick enough to be in a hospital Intensive Care Unit (*ICU*)

Many healthy consumers use various probiotic products assuming that the probiotics will help maintain and promote their health by reducing the long-term risk of various diseases. However, although healthy people are the common target for these new functional or super food products, the number of clinical trials proving effectiveness have been quite limited even though many research studies are underway. In one sense, unless products are available, there is nothing to take or to test clinically; yet on the other hand, when there is a plethora of products calling themselves probiotics that are not clinically proven, the consumer or health care provider is unsure which to take and what to expect from their use. But research and molecular science is compiling a lot of good helpful information every year.

• http://www.ncbi.nlm.nih.gov/books/NBK56091/pdf/TOC.pdf

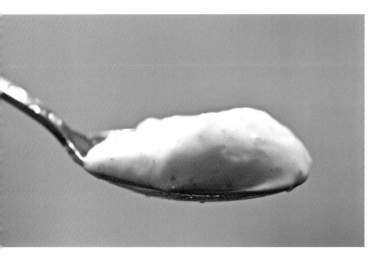

Chapter 6
NAMES OF THE MOST COMMON PROBIOTIC MICROBES

B= Bifidobacterium L = Lactobacillus S = Saccharomyces

The following are the most common probiotic strains for readers' understanding/information only. This list may not be fully inclusive.

- B. brevis
- B. longus
- B. lactis
- Bacillus species
- Enterococcus species
- Escherichia coli nissle 1917 - was one of the first probiotics to be used
- L. acidophilus
- L. amylovorus
- L. brevis
- L. bulgaricus
- L. casei
- L. casei immunitas
- L. crispatus
- L. delbrueckii
- L. fermentum
- L. gallinarum
- L. helveticus
- L. johnsonii
- L. lactis
- L. plantarum
- L. reuteri
- L. rhamnosus
- L. salivarius
- L. paracasei
- L. sakei
- L. sporogenes
- Leuconostoc cremoris
- S. boulardii
- S. diacetylactis
- S. florentinus
- Streptococcus thermophilus

The commercial probiotic yogurt Activia® has a proprietary probiotic strain *Bifidus regularis* (*commercial name*). The true name of this probiotic is *Bifidobacterium lactis DN 173010*. The commonly available health food supplement **kefir** has multiple strains of probiotics: *L. reuteri, L. casei, L. lactis, L.acidophilus, L. rhamnosus, L.plantarum, Leuconostoc cremoris, S. diacetylactis, S. florentinus, Bifidobacterium lactis, B. longus, B. brevis.* There are numerous probiotic health foods in the market these days. After you take a probiotic, the DNA of the probiotic strain is detectable on your colon lining. The probiotics do not inhabit your gut permanently. After you stop taking the supplement, they typically disappear from the gut within a few weeks.

The next time you are at the supermarket read the label and try to identify the probiotics.

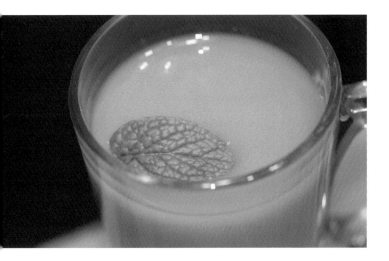

Chapter 7
COMMON PROBIOTIC FOODS

THERE ARE CERTAIN FOODS THAT NATURALLY HAVE PROBIOTICS IN THEM. Probiotic foods can be dairy and non-dairy. Dairy-based foods include yogurt, buttermilk, kefir (*dairy based*) and other animal (*cow, goat, donkey*) milk-based products. Non-dairy foods include soy foods and beverages, vegetable or fruit-based (*coconut*) fermented foods, tempeh, miso, sauerkraut, soft cheeses, kimbucha tea, kimchi, bean ferment and non-dairy kefir.

Kefir is a fermented milk drink made with kefir "grains" (*a yeast/ bacterial fermentation starter*) and has its origins in the north Caucasus Mountains around 3000 B.C. Kefir can be made from cow milk, goat milk and coconut milk. Kefir has multiple strains of bacteria namely *Lactobacillus, Bifidobacterium, Leuconostoc cremaris* and *Saccharomyces* (*yeast*).

Probiotics also occur naturally in certain traditional Japanese foods such as **miso**, a seasoning prepared by fermenting rice, barley and soybeans with salt and yeast. Miso has abundant *Lactobacilli*. **Miso** can also be prepared from pistachios, pine nuts, lentils or mung beans. Nut-based **misos** have a sweet and creamy delicious taste.

Sauerkraut is fermented cabbage with salt, water and *Lactobacillus* species. **Bean ferment** is typically made with red beans soaked in water. Then, the water is poured away, and onions, garlic, cabbage and tomato brine from sauerkraut are added. It also has an abundance of *Lactobacilli*. **Tempeh** is a fermented Indonesian soy cake with fungus *Rhizopus* species.

Kimchi is a spicy, fiery, fermented Korean dish made with onion, garlic, ginger, cabbage and hot pepper. It is rich in *Lactobacilli*. **Balao-balao** is a Filipino specialty in which rice is fermented with shrimp with action of *Lactobacilli*.

Soft cheeses are one of the most popular gourmet fermented foods and are a big pillar of the food industry. They are rich in *Lactococcus, Lactobacilli and Streptococci*. Little needs to be said about **Sourdough bread**, born in San Francisco, California, with its simply awesome flavor. It is also easy to digest and is well tolerated by people with celiac disease.

In the Indian subcontinent, vegetables and fruits such as raw mangoes, lemons, ginger and other food items are pickled using salt, vinegar and *Lactobacillus* culture starters. This provides storage for excess food, hence minimizing food wastage. These pickles serve as flavor enhancing sides to gourmet Indian cuisine.

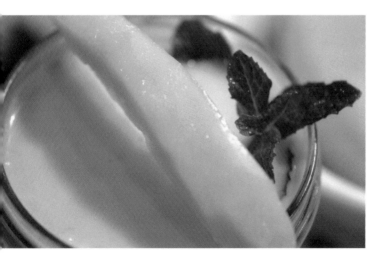

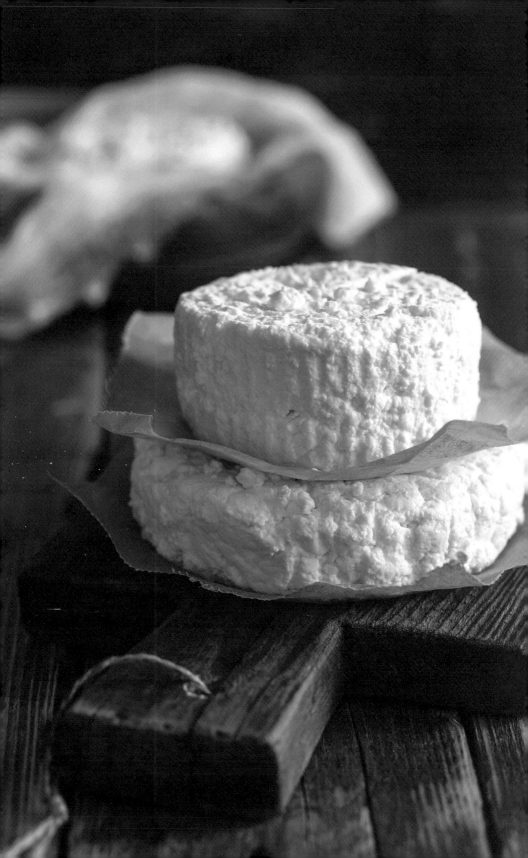

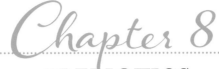

Chapter 8
PREBIOTICS:
Food for the Good Bacteria

PREBIOTICS PROVIDE THE FERTILE SOIL FOR PROLIFERATION OF PROBIOTICS. We have to be careful not to confuse the prebiotics with probiotics. *Prebiotics* are *Non-Digestible Oligo Saccharides (NDOS)* or simply short chain carbohydrates that are selectively broken down by the gut bacteria and serve as their food. Hence, by providing certain foods or mixtures with NDOS, we can promote growth of good bacteria and the associated health benefits.

They can selectively trigger growth of certain beneficial types of bacteria such as *Lactobacilli* and *Bifidobacteria,* which then interact with the immune system and bring about the changes in immune status and health. Prebiotics are the agents or food components that basically feed the good bacteria and enhance their populability. Prebiotics are small chains of carbohydrates (*e.g. fructose, galactose*).

Common prebiotics are either fructo-oligosaccharides, polymers of fructose or galacto-oligosaccharides, polymers of galactose. Most prebiotics are plant storage carbohydrates. They are found in wheat, onion, bananas, garlic, asparagus and chicory. Prebiotics have no effect on metabolism or absorption of other nutrients, but they do help to lower the pH of the colon.

Fiber carbohydrates such as cellulose are fermented into short chain fatty acids in the lower gastrointestinal tract due to lack of bacterial/enzymatic capability and may promote growth of certain good bacteria. Thus, diet can change the type of bacteria that colonize your gut because bacteria feed on certain energy sources to thrive.

Today, only inulin, and its breakdown product oligo-fructose and (*trans*) galacto-oligosaccharides, fulfill all the criteria for prebiotic classification. It has a well-established positive impact on the intestinal microflora, especially growth of *Bifidobacterium*.

Certain food products contain a prebiotics and probiotics combination. They are known as synbiotics. Pectin is a soluble fiber and is considered a good prebiotic. Apples, citrus fruit rinds, crab apples, cranberries, currants, gooseberries, plums and grapes are rich sources of pectin.

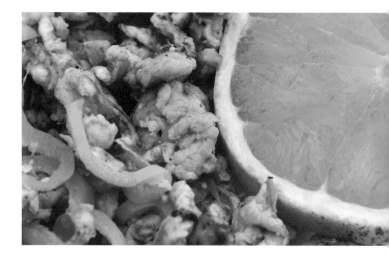

This table illustrates prebiotics and some medical conditions they have been studied in. This is NOT a treatment recommendation.

PREBIOTIC	MEDICAL CONDITION*
Inulin	Crohn's disease, Colitis, Obesity, Type 2 Diabetes, Colon cancer, Constipation
FOS (*Fructo-oligosaccharides*)	Crohn's disease, Colitis, Obesity, Traveler's diarrhea, Colon cancer, Constipation
GOS (*Galacto-oligosaccharides*)	Crohn's disease, Colitis, Obesity
Soluble fiber (*Guar gum, pectin*)	Crohn's disease, Colitis, Obesity, Metabolic syndrome, Arthritis, Colon cancer, Cardiovascular diseases

* These are the medical conditions the above mentioned prebiotics are studied in. Based on the available clinical and medical literature, the effectiveness is variable. *See References on page 61.*

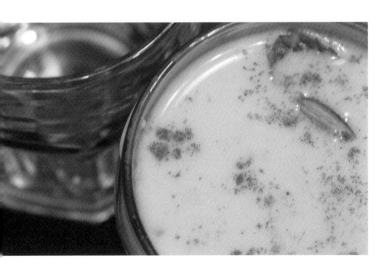

Chapter 9

ROLE OF PROBIOTICS:
Health Benefits

WE ALREADY KNOW THAT PROBIOTICS CAN PROMOTE GOOD HEALTH. Some research studies have shown a role for probiotics in shortening the symptom duration for certain gastrointestinal conditions such as *Clostridium difficile* infection, which results due to use (*over use*) of antibiotics to treat infections. Antibiotics kill the good bacteria, hence paving way for *C. difficile* infection. It is detected by Polymerase Chain Reaction (*PCR*) technology-based testing of stool sample, which could be either delivered to the lab by the patient or collected by colonoscopy by the gastroenterologist.

Tens of millions of dollars are spent every year for medical treatment of *C. difficile* associated infection and hospitalization. There are many new medications on the market for treatment, but *C. difficile* is a demon that resulted from antibiotic overuse in the 21st century. Probiotics may have a role in *Clostridium difficile* Associated Diarrhea (*CDAD*). Probiotics also have a role in Antibiotic Associated Diarrhea (*AAD*), which results from the (*over*) use of antibiotics creating an imbalance in the gut microbiota and may cause debilitating diarrhea, abdominal cramps and discomfort. This needs to be differentiated from *C. difficile* diarrhea. *C. difficile* may recur after treatment and is becoming a major problem.

Another condition affecting about 53 million Americans is Irritable Bowel Syndrome, or IBS. It presents as abdominal pain, bloating, change in bowel habits, which could be either constipation or diarrhea.

Increasing evidence is again hinting toward gut bacteria's dominant role in IBS pathophysiology. A recent human study has shown that the probiotic *Lactobacillus acidophilus* species actually calms down some of the pain receptors in the human gut known as Mu receptors. This helps minimize pain in IBS. IBS also needs to be distinguished from Small Bowel Bacterial Overgrowth Syndrome, a condition where "bad bacteria" overgrow in your small bowel and can cause IBS-like symptoms. Rarely, diseases of carbohydrate malabsorption, where certain carbohydrates like fructose and lactose cannot be absorbed from the diet, can cause symptoms similar to IBS. Please discuss these symptoms with your health care provider and do not self diagnose or treat.

Another set of disease driven by your immune system is IBD or Inflammatory Bowel Disease. IBD is NOT IBS. IBD has been proposed to result from "disharmony" between your immune system and the gut microbes, hence it has received major interest from the probiotic manufacturers. IBD has two main subtypes: Ulcerative Colitis and Crohn's disease. There is medical literature supporting the notion that gut microbiota has a tremendous role in IBD manifestation. There is complex interaction and cross talk between your gut bacteria and immune system that is overseen by your genetic risk factors. The only probiotic that has shown good benefit in Ulcerative Colitis and Pouchitis is VSL #3®. Culturelle and Florastor have been studied in Crohn's disease, but no clear benefit has been seen so far and more research is needed. About 2.5 billion CFU a day are beneficial in IBS. As per a recent study, at least 6.5 billion CFUs of probiotic were needed to be helpful against infectious diarrhea. Technically speaking, a higher dose and multiple microbes will be preferred over single strain and lesser number of CFUs. Let's discuss briefly a few products. Culturelle® has 10 billion CFUs of Lactobacillus GG while Align® has 1 billion CFUs of

Bifidobacterium. BioK+® has about 12.5 billion - 50 billion CFUs per capsule. Every manufacturer is different but a minimum 1-2 billion CFUs is necessary to get benefit. Higher dose and multiple microbes will be preferred over single strain and less amount. But please do discuss with your doctor any time you will be increasing the dose of the probiotic or taking a certain type of probiotic. New research pours in everyday; hence, the dose and type of beneficial probiotic is a moving target.

The table below lays out the commercial probiotic products, available in USA, Canada, Europe and Asia. I have also mentioned the medical conditions those probiotics can potentially target based on current evidence.

AVAILABLE PROBIOTIC PRODUCTS
Specifically Tested for Gastrointestinal Disorders

ACRONYMS:
AAD-Antibiotic Associated Diarrhea
CDAD-Clostridium Difficile Associated Diarrhea

COMMERCIAL PRODUCT *Probiotic strains*	MEDICAL CONDITION *(Tested in)* *Variable effectiveness based on clinical evidence/medical literature*
Activia® *B. lactis, L. bulgaricus, L. lactis, S. thermophilus* http://www.danone.com	Irritable Bowel Synrome (IBS)
Align® *B. infantis* http://www.aligngi.com	Irritable Bowel Synrome (IBS)
Actimel/Danactive® *L. casei* http://www.danone.com	AAD prevention, CDAD prevention, ID prevention

Continues on pages 31-32.

COMMERCIAL PRODUCT *Probiotic strains*	MEDICAL CONDITION *(Tested in)* *Variable effectiveness based on clinical* *evidence/medical literature*
BioGaia® *L. reuteri Protectis* www.biokplus.com	IBS, ID treatment
BioK +® *L. acidophilus, L. casei* www.biokplus.com	AAD prevention, CDAD prevention
Culturelle® *Lactobacillus casei subsp.* *Rhamnosus GG* www.valio.com	AAD prevention, CDAD prevention, ID treatment and prevention, Crohn's disease, IBS, prevention of rotavirus-related diarrhea in children, reduces the risk of respiratory tract infections in children, useful in the prevention of atopic dermatitis in children at high risk of allergy
Enterogermina® *Bacillus clausii* en.sanofi.com	Reduces adverse effects and increases tolerability of Helicobacter Pylori eradication therapy, Allergic Rhinitis in children
Mutaflor® *ECN Escherichia Coli Nissle 1917* www.ardeypharm.de/en/	Inflammatory Bowel Disease, IBS, acute diarrhea, chronic constipation
Miyarisan® *Clostridium butyricum MIYAIRI588* www.miyarisan.com	Antibiotic-associated diarrhea, reduction of side effects of H. Pylori treatment

COMMERCIAL PRODUCT *Probiotic strains*	MEDICAL CONDITION *(Tested in)* *Variable effectiveness based on clinical evidence/medical literature*
Probio-Tec® *Bifidobacterium animalis subsp. Lactis BB-12Chr* www.chr-hansen.com	Relieves constipation, improves fecal properties and microbiota, has positive effects against acute diarrhea, reduces antibiotic-associated diarrhea, enhances the intestinal antibody response in formula-fed infants
VSL #3® *Streptococcus thermophilus, B. breve, B. longum, B. infantis, L. acidophilus, L. plantarum, L. paracasei, L. delbreuckii/bulgaricus* www.sigmatau.com	IBS, Ulcerative Colitis *(induction and maintenance),* Pouchitis *(inflammation of ileal pouch after colectomy for UC),* prevention and maintaining remission
Ultra-levure® **(Florastor)** *Saccharomyces boulardii (yeast)* www.biocodex.com	AAD prevention, CDAD prevention, ID treatment and prevention, CDAD prevention of recurrence, Crohn's disease *(needs more clinical evidence)*
Yakult® *Lactobacillus casei shirota* www.yakult.co.jp/english/	AAD prevention, Infectious diarrhea treatment and prevention, CDAD prevention, CDAD prevention of recurrence, Crohn's disease *(needs more clinical evidence)*

Source - *Please see References 1 and 2 on page 61.*

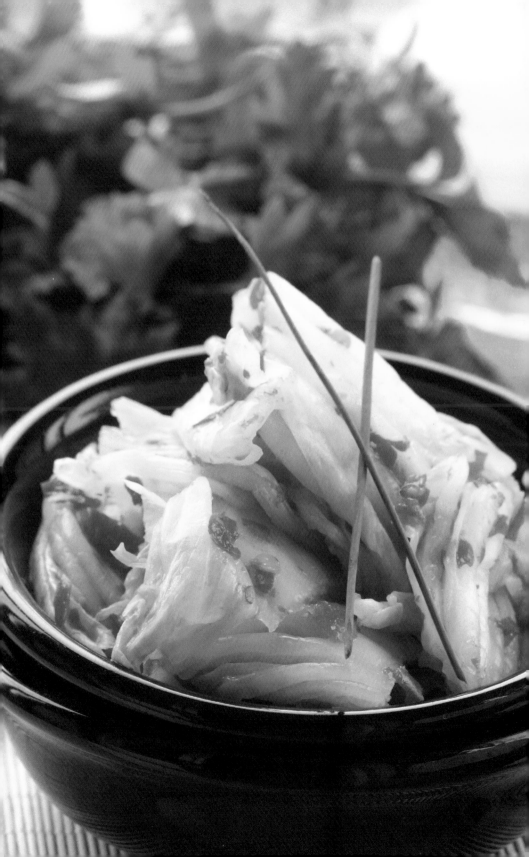

Chapter 10
WHAT ELSE IS ON
THE HORIZON?

THE NEXT DECADE WILL BRING MORE ADVANCES.

Probiotics are being investigated to clarify their impact on:

1. Mood disorders

2. Chronic Fatigue Syndrome

3. Irritable Bowel Syndrome

4. Obesity and Metabolic Syndrome

5. Autism

6. Inflammatory Bowel Disease

7. Asthma and allergies

In animal models, probiotics have been assesed for benefit against radiation injury. Research is also underway to identify specific soluble factors or products of metabolism from the probiotics. They can potentially be isolated and then sold as a concentrated product. This would be ideal!

Another novel probiotic is *Enterococcus faecium IS 27526*. It is isolated from dadih, an Indonesian traditional fermented buffalo milk. A study conducted on preschool children to assess the beneficial effects of dadih showed elevation in Total IgA antibody level in the saliva as well as increase in body weight.

Researchers are investigating how *Lactobacillus species* (*Lactobacillus reuteri ATCC PTA 6475*) might work to slow the growth of certain cancerous tumors. They are trying to unmask the molecular mechanism that regulates the proliferation of cancer cells and promotes cancer cell death. A better understanding of these effects may lead to development of probiotic-based regimens to prevent colorectal cancer, urogenital cancer and Inflammatory Bowel Disease.

Lactobacillus acidophilus has been evaluated to enhance the immune-potentiating effects of an attenuated vaccine (*a vaccine prepared from a weakened live virus*) against human rotavirus infection — the most common cause of severe dehydrating diarrhea in infants and children worldwide. In animal studies, scientists have discovered that animals given both a vaccine and the probiotic had a better immune response than the animals given the vaccine alone. Thus, probiotics may offer a safe way to potentiate the effectiveness of rotavirus vaccine in humans.

Probiotics have been extensively investigated to reduce colic in infants. Probiotics are being added to infant formula feeds. A recent pediatric study published in the Journal of the American Medical Association (JAMA) states that the use of probiotic *L. Reuteri DSM 17938* during the first 3 months of life reduced the onset of colic, regurgitation and functional constipation in children. This may help us save millions of health care dollars.

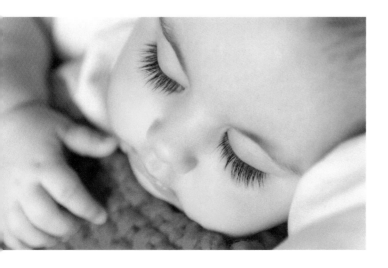

Chapter 11

PROBIOTIC GASTRONOMY:
Fermented Foods

GAS·TRON·O·MY: THE ART OR ACTIVITY OF COOKING AND EATING FINE FOOD. Gastronomy follows basic scientific principles that support the methodology of cooking, food preparation and the enjoyment of food. The Food Science and Technology industry appreciates the scientific basis of various recipes, and focuses on developing new recipes by integrating the scientific principles into new dishes. They recognize the influence of human perception from the different senses and try to integrate science into cooking and dining. The science of fermentation can help chefs and food scientists channel their creative energies through discovery of new foods and flavors.

Humans learned to enjoy fermented foods a long time ago. It started with the elegant mastery of fermenting wheat, corn and fruits into alcoholic beverages, which is gastronomically and financially a billion dollar industry. The science of fermentation has evolved across all cultures over many centuries. Food technology and food science are constantly making progress toward enhancing food flavors. Microbes have played a key role in the explosive evolution of cuisines due to flavor enhancement. The aromas and flavors are invigorating for the soul.

The activities of these microbial communities lend distinctive flavors, textures and aromas to fermented foods, which appears to vary from region to region. Restaurants have research and development divisions that experiment with different foods and microbes to enhance the flavor.

TASTE RECEPTORS ARE THE END CLIENTELE OF ALL FOOD FLAVORS

The microbes are our friends and have unfailingly catered to our taste buds. Realistically, human taste receptors are the end clientele of all food flavors. Taste buds contain the receptors for taste sensation. The highest concentration of taste buds is in the small elevations known as "protuberances" on the tongue. These are called "papillae." Each taste bud has about 100 receptors that are called "neuroepithelial receptors" meaning it's a lining that is connected to a nerve fibre to carry the taste signal to the brain.

Most of the taste signals travel through the 7, 9 and 10 cranial nerves (*facial, glossopharyngeal and vagus, respectively*) to reach the taste and smell area of the brain for further signal processing.

There are five primary qualities of taste:

1. **Sweet** (*signal presence of carbohydrates, which provide energy*)
2. **Sour** (*presence of dietary acids*)
3. **Salty** (*this sensation helps to regulate body water, salt balance and blood pressure*)
4. **Bitter** (*aversive and is a protective evolutionary sensation against ingestion of poisons*)
5. **Umami or savory** (*reflects protein content of food L glutamic acid and L-amino acids*). Umami is the target of MSG, the commercial food flavoring product.

Here I should mention Professor Kikunae Ikeda, a Japanese chemist and Tokyo Imperial University chemistry professor, who in 1908 (*same year when Elie Metchnikoff received the Nobel Prize for his work on Phagocytosis: defense mechanism for destroying pathogens*) uncovered the chemical root behind a taste he named umami, which is one of the five basic tastes along with sweet, bitter, sour and salty. He discovered that the common component that produced the flavor of meat, seaweed and tomatoes was glutamate, which produces the sensation of umami, or savoriness. He patented the manufacture of monosodium glutamate.

There are a lot of health concerns about MSG's safety, but in November 2012 the FDA released their position statement on their website stating that there is not enough information to deem MSG a health risk.

- http://www.fda.gov/food/ingredientspackaginglabeling/foodadditives ingredients/ucm328728.htm

Some people may have headaches, migraines, palpitations and some other vague symptoms after MSG ingestion. Please follow the link below if you want to learn more. It is beyond the scope of this book to get into the details of MSG side effects. The FDA shall have the final authority over this.

The science of fermentation has been known for ages, yet it is still evolving. Fermentation has widely expanded the spectrum of what's available to the human taste buds. Fermented foods offer complex and irresistible flavors. When combined with a probiotic or good bacterial health boost we will have a "super food." Fermented cheeses, miso, koji, sauerkraut, sourdough bread (*making San Francisco proud*), kimchi, tempeh, soy sauce and tamari (*a soy sauce like Japanese sauce made from fermented soy that has less wheat, less sodium and has more amino acids*) are some examples of gourmet fermented foods.

Restaurant owners utilize the art of fermentation as one of their tools to enhance flavors. It is equivalent to a food chemistry lab where the end product is creative gourmet food for total indulgence. The products of microbial metabolism help modulate or change the activity of enzymes in the food which, in turn, offer substrate or raw material for bacterial growth, functioning as an ecosystem. Food technologists and restaurateurs use DNA sequencing to detect the microbial species (*fungi and bacteria*) present in their food. According to a prominent Harvard microbiologist/food scientist, Dr. Rachel Dutton, 90 percent of the world's sourdough contains a single species of bacteria: *Lactobacillus sanfranciscensis*. So if you want to reproduce the flavor or consistency you can target this microbe to make your starter culture. It is equivalent to having a fingerprint or a DNA sample to trace back the microbial origin of a particular taste.

It is very risky to harvest and utilize the microbes to your benefit. Skilled personnel with access to a sophisticated scientific lab, specialized equipment and a controlled environment are needed. There are companies that will provide research and scientific support to individuals or companies interested in manufacturing probiotic food products. I do not recommend or endorse attempts to create or consume complex fermented foods for personal use. The future of probiotic gastronomy will be bright and flavorful.

PROBIOTIC
Recipes

"To keep the body in good health
is a duty, for otherwise we shall not
be able to trim the lamp of wisdom,
and keep our mind strong and clear.
Water surrounds the lotus flower,
but does not wet its petals."

– BUDDHA

**I AM LISTING SOME EASY RECIPES THAT I HAVE TRIED
MYSELF AND FOUND TO BE HELPFUL.** At this time I am not going
into detail of how to make your own probiotic foods. This is not pertinent
to the message of this book. For the purpose of making it easy on readers
and ensuring good quality food product we will use the readily available
ingredients from local grocery stores. I would like to take this opportunity
to counsel against the consumption of alcoholic beverages and/or
tobacco products. Always pick products with low trans fat and low salt.
In the case of precooked products, I recommend baked over fried.

These recipes do not replace medical advice from your health care
provider. Please do not consume any fermented foods if you suspect they
might be spoiled or if you have a serious illness or health issues.

If you have diabetes, heart disease, high blood pressure or other
illnessess, please speak with your health care provider before you try
any of these recipes. If you are pregnant, lactating or planning to be pregnant,
please talk to your health care provider before you try any of these recipes.

STRAWBERRY FIRE: KEFIR BASED SMOOTHIE

LOVE IS A SPIRIT ALL COMPACT OF FIRE

8 to 10 oz. non-flavored low fat kefir

25 blueberries, *frozen or fresh*

10 strawberries, *frozen or fresh*

10 grams fresh cut ginger root for the spicy aftertaste
May use ginger powder if needed

1. Blend all these ingredients in an electric blender.
   May add 4-5 ice cubes. Crush them into a smoothie.

2. May garnish with a sprinkle of cinnamon powder
   or a fresh mint leaf to get a summer feel.

Drink either alone or as part of a meal. Enjoy the probiotic, antioxidant boost. Ginger will offer the zing or fire taste. In Ayurveda, ginger is a medicinal herb useful in cold and flu illnesses. Ginger also causes some dilation of the blood vessels, enhancing blood flow to hands and feet.

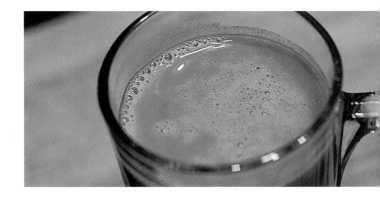

HE LOVES ME, HE LOVES ME "NUTS"

KEFIR OR GREEK YOGURT BASED SMOOTHIE

8 to 10 oz. non-flavored low fat kefir

or 5 oz. of low fat or low fat Greek yogurt

If you use Greek yogurt you will need to dilute with water
or low-fat milk. The nuts will make the smoothie thick and creamy

10 almonds, *cleaned and soaked*

10 pecans

5 cashews, *adds a creamy taste*

2 walnuts

1/2 cup mango slices

1. Blend all these ingredients in an electric blender.
   May add 4-5 ice cubes. Crush into a smoothie.

2. May garnish with a sprinkle of cinnamon powder
   or a hint of ginger extract.

This drink will be very creamy, so you may want to dilute. Drink
either alone or as part of a meal. Enjoy the probiotic, antioxidant boost
plus protein boost. A memory boosting drink. Nuts are a good source
of Omega-3 fatty acids for heart, brain and eyes, as well as fiber,
Vitamin E and L-arginine, which helps against building of plaque in
your arteries.

VENUS AND ADONIS: FRUIT BOOST

It's called Venus and Adonis because this drink is pretty.
It's an elixir of love and passion.

1 cup low-fat, non-flavored kefir or buttermilk

1/2 cup peaches, *freshly peeled and cut*

1/4 cup passion fruit pulp

1/2 cup mango pulp

10 fresh blueberries, *washed*

8 raspberries, *frozen or fresh*

8 almonds

1. Blend all these ingredients until smooth in an electric blender.

2. Add low-fat whipped cream in a swirl.

Enjoy this pretty drink with a loved one *(or alone, if you love thyself more and don't like sharing)*. If it gets too sweet you may want to complement the flavor with something salty on the side, such as a few salted cashews or crackers!

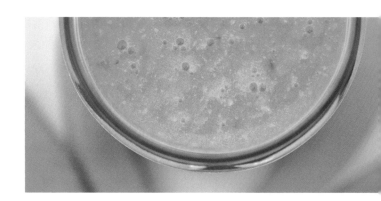

TANGY "PUNJAB" MANGO BUTTERMILK

Experience the flavors that the hard-working farmers of Northern Indian state of Punjab *(land of five rivers)* enjoy daily. Either you can buy a brand from the store or make your own. There are a lot of good online resources to make buttermilk at home.

2 cups buttermilk

1/2 cup ripe mangoes or mango pulp
(preserved pulp will have higher sugar content)

1/4 teaspoon cardamom powder

5 mint leaves, *optional*

1. Blend with ice cubes.

2. Garnish with 5 minced fresh mint leaves.

Serve chilled and feel the refreshing breeze from the farms of Punjab. Locally it is called lassi and is part of the staple diet.

OH "SO COOL" AND SIMPLE BUTTERMILK

The locals of Punjab drink buttermilk by the gallons during hot summer months.

2 cups of low-fat buttermilk

5 mint leaves

fresh water

black pepper and table salt

1. Blend the buttermilk with 5 mint leaves and 4-5 ice cubes. May add water according to your preference for thickness.

2. Sprinkle a pinch of table salt and a pinch of black pepper — Drink it like a champ!

YOU CALLIN' ME CUMIN?

2 cups buttermilk or non-flavored kefir

1/4 teaspoon of cumin powder

1/8 teaspoon of black pepper

table salt according to taste

oregano, *fresh or dried*

1. Blend buttermilk with cumin, black pepper, salt with 4-5 ice cubes. May need to add water to dilute.

2. Garnish with some oregano — Enjoy!

SOAK IN THE MONSOON: TROPICAL DELIGHT

2 cups buttermilk or low-fat, non-flavored kefir

1 tablespoon shaved coconut pulp

1 oz. coconut milk

5 strawberries, *fresh cut or frozen*

1 oz. pineapple, *fresh*

mint leaves, *optional*

1. Blend the above ingredients with ice.

2. May garnish with fresh mint leaves.

Pour into glass and savor the flavors. With each sip let the fresh, clean and cool tropical monsoon breeze blow your mind away. Best place to enjoy this would be on the beach on a hot summer day!

BUTTERMILK CILANTRO MINT DIP

1/2 cup of buttermilk
May add some probiotic Greek yogurt to the dip to thicken it

15 fresh cilantro leaves, *rinsed*

8 fresh mint leaves *(or according to taste)*

1/4 teaspoon salt

5 drops of vinegar

1/4 teaspoon garlic powder

1/4 teaspoon cumin powder

1 small sun dried tomato

1/4 teaspoon of low-fat mayonnaise

1/8 teaspoon black pepper

Blend all the above ingredients. May add some water to dilute.

This is an all-purpose dip and is my personal favorite. It's a frenzy of flavors. Enjoy this with vegetables, chicken wings or finger foods of choice. This is better than ranch or other dressings that might have a lot of unhealthy fat, artificial flavors or preservatives.

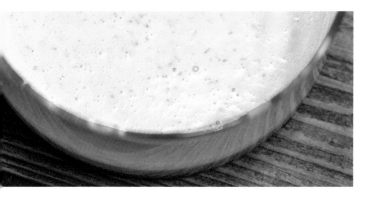

PACK A FOUR LAYERED PUNCH, THE "KNOCK OUT" BREAKFAST BOWL

2 cups crispy oatmeal granola cereal

1/2 cup chopped or sliced almonds

1/2 cup chopped walnuts

1/2 cup dried cranberries

1/4 cup chopped pistachios

1/2 cup fresh peaches or canned peaches
(strain off the extra syrup)

1/2 cup flavored Greek yogurt

1. For the first layer, pour the granola cereal into a bowl.

2. For the second layer, add the almonds, walnuts, cranberries and pistachios.

3. For the third layer, add peaches or your fresh fruit of choice.

4. The fourth layer will be of delicious yogurt.

Enjoy this with fresh orange juice or kefir drink! Perfect way to overcome early morning mental inertia with healthy carbohydrate, fiber, good fatty acids, protein, vitamins and probiotic boost.

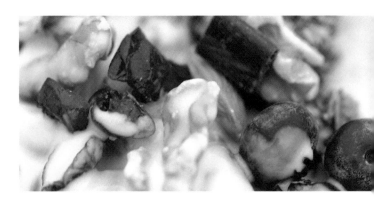

SCRAMBLE OF COLORS: WHICH CAME FIRST, THE CITRUS OR THE EGG?

Another of my favorites. Scrambled egg, vegetables, with grapefruit. Yum!

3 whole large chicken eggs
(lighter option: replace with 5 egg whites)

1/3 cup red bell pepper

1/3 cup yellow bell pepper

1/3 cup diced tomatoes, *fresh*

1/3 cup red onions

1/4 cup green onions

1 green chili

1/2 cup olive oil

1 grapefruit

1 glass buttermilk or low-fat kefir or
low-fat yogurt smoothie with active cultures

1. Heat 1/2 cup of olive oil in a non-stick pan.

2. Break and beat 3 whole eggs. Pour the eggs into the pan and stir/ scramble. *(If you have high cholesterol issues, please use egg white only)*

3. Add the chopped vegetables. Stir the mixture till egg turns golden brown.

4. Add salt according to taste, preferably low salt. Optional: add fresh green chili, just enough for the color and spice. Cook for 5 -10 minutes on medium heat. Do not overcook the vegetables or the eggs.

Garnish with fresh cilantro, green onions and 2 slices of fresh grapefruit on the side. Experience the Vitamin C, probiotic, healthy protein, antioxidant boost along with the unsaturated fatty acids from olive oil. Enjoy this with flavored kefir or buttermilk.

HEAVEN AND EARTH: COCONUT BUTTERMILK WAFFLES WITH GREEK YOGURT

3 cups whole wheat flour

1/4 cup of flax seeds, *powdered*

3 large eggs

1/4 cup coconut milk

1 cup low-fat buttermilk

1/2 cup olive oil

1 tablespoon of sugar

1 teaspoon table salt

3/4 teaspoon baking soda

Mix all the dry ingredients into a batter. Pour this into wafflemaker and follow standard instructions for making waffles.

Top the waffles with Greek yogurt or other active culture yogurt, fresh blueberries and strawberries. Pour low-calorie maple syrup or regular syrup. Enjoy with your choice of drink: sweet kefir or sweetened buttermilk. Soy milk or almond milk will also complement these waffles and send your taste buds into a euphoric frenzy.

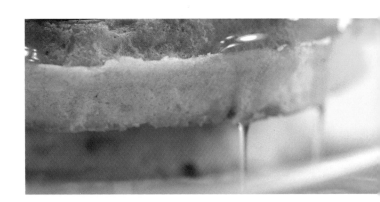

RENDER UNTO CAESAR THAT IS WHICH IS CAESAR'S: HEALTHY SALAD WITH PROBIOTIC DRESSING

1/2 pound lettuce, *fresh cut*

2 large fresh tomatoes, *sliced and diced*

1/4 pound spinach

10 baby carrots, *sliced*

1/4 cup green string beans

1/4 red onion, *cut into long thin slices*

2 cucumbers, *peeled and diced*

6-8 dried cranberries

1 oz. buttermilk with active cultures or non-flavored low fat kefir

1 teaspoon lemon juice

1/4 teaspoon of basil powder

1/4 teaspoon of olive oil

1/4 teaspoon of almond oil

1/4 teaspoon of oregano powder

sea salt, *to taste*

1. Prepare the dressing by mixing buttermilk/kefir, basil powder, olive oil, almond oil, lemon juice, oregano powder and salt in a blender or bowl. This is a low-fat delicious dressing.

2. Mix all the vegetables in a large salad bowl. Pour the dressing over the greens and enjoy.

This is a healthier choice over ranch or heavy duty fat dressings. Get a good fiber and probiotic boost!

CUCUMBER & BROCCOLI DIP

2 cups low-fat unsweetened kefir

1/2 cup cucumber, *fresh cut*

1/2 cup broccoli, *rinsed and steamed until soft*

6-8 mint leaves

5-8 basil leaves

10 cilantro leaves

2 teaspoons olive oil

1/4 teaspoon oregano

sea salt, *to taste*

Blend all the above ingredients together into a paste. Add salt according to taste.

Now you have a cool cucumber broccoli dip. Enjoy this with baked low-carb corn chips or your choice of fresh cut or baked vegetables.

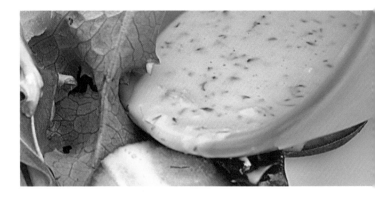

SPINACH, TOFU AND MISO SOUP: JAPANESE DELIGHT

1/2 cup baby spinach leaves

1/2 cup tofu, *medium diced*

2 tablespoons miso *(preferably red or brown)*
Miso paste is available at local grocery stores

1/4 cup onion greens

1 tablespoon sesame oil

1-2 tablespoons tamari sauce

1. In a pan, heat up sesame oil on low heat and then add spinach, green onions and tofu. Stir for about 1 min.

2. In a separate small bowl, mix 2 tablespoons miso paste with 1 cup boiling water to dissolve.

3. Add the stirred vegetables to the soup. Use tamari sauce for extra flavor.

Better served hot. Pour into a soup bowl and enjoy the soy protein and probiotic boost.

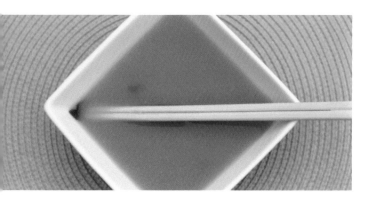

MEATBALLS WITH SAUERKRAUT

**32 oz. frozen precooked chicken, turkey or beef meatballs
(1 full package-*preferably low fat, white meat*)**

1 can cranberry sauce

1/2 teaspoon of paprika

1/2 cup of brown sugar

1 cup sauerkraut, *well rinsed and drained*

1/4 cup non-flavored kefir

In a slow cooker (or crock pot) mix the meatballs, cranberry sauce, brown sugar, non-flavored kefir and sauerkraut. Cover the lid and slowly cook for 5-6 hours till well cooked.

Enjoy with a citrus based drink such as lemonade or orange juice or tangy salted buttermilk to offset the sweet flavor of the dish. The sauerkraut works great as a side dish as well. *Caution: This dish may not be suitable for people with diabetes, high blood pressure or heart disease.*

SAUERKRAUT AND SAUSAGE

1 cup sauerkraut, *well rinsed and drained*

2-3 Chicken, turkey or beef sausages

1/3 red onion, *sliced and diced*

Condiments: *relish, mustard and or ketchup*

You can either grill or boil the sausages till well done.

Use whole wheat hot dog buns. Garnish with condiments, onion, coriander and sauerkraut. Enjoy with kefir drink or buttermilk.

QUICKIE KIMCHI: KIMCHI IN A HURRY

A Korean meal is not complete without kimchi. Traditional Korean families used to prepare enough kimchi to last the long winter. The kimchi was stored in large clay jars that were partially buried to maintain temperature to enhance fermentation and retain flavor. Kimchi is a delicious mixture of various pickled vegetables, such as cabbage, radish, green onion and cucumber with red chili pepper and garlic for more flavor.

1 cup premade kimchi *(buy from local grocery or Asian market)*

1/2 cup sesame oil

1 cup precooked diced chicken

1/2 cup tofu

Stir-fry kimchi in sesame oil in pan. Add diced chicken, tofu and water. Cook until the meat is tender. Then serve with brown or white rice. Alternatively, just eat it as is.

Caution: Some people may not like the acidic fermented taste of kimchi. Kimchi also has a lot of sodium that is not good for people with heart, liver or kidney disease.

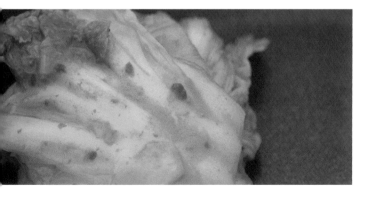

SCRAMBLED EGGS WITH SAUTÉED KIMCHI

1 cup premade kimchi (*buy from local grocery or Asian market*)

1/2 cup sesame oil

1/2 tablespoon tamari sauce

3 whole eggs or 5 egg whites

1/4 cup bell peppers, *chopped and diced*

1/4 red onion, *chopped*

1 tomato, *chopped and diced*

cilantro leaves to garnish

Heat sesame oil in a pan. Add kimchi sautee until it develops a caramelized finish. Add eggs and scramble till well done. Top with fresh diced vegetables.

May enjoy with whole wheat toast and buttermilk or kefir.

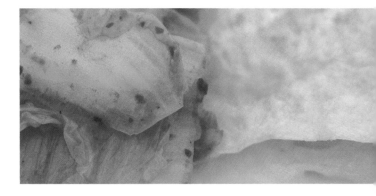

AWESOME GUACAMOLE DIP

1/2 cup non-flavored kefir or buttermilk

2 avocados, chopped

2 tomatoes

1/2 red onion, *chopped*

2 green chili peppers, *finely chopped*

8-10 mint leaves, *finely chopped*

10-15 cilantro leaves, *finely chopped*

1/2 teaspoon lime juice

sea salt, *to taste*

1 packet guacamole seasoning

baked pita bread or baked corn tortillas

Add avocados, red onion, chopped green peppers, mint leaves and cilantro into a bowl and mix well. Add the kefir or buttermilk. Squeeze 1/2 teaspoon of lime juice into the mixture. Add some guacamole seasoning. Mix well. Bake pita bread at 350 degrees in the oven for 10-15 mins. The end result should be crispy bread that can be cut into chips.

Enjoy with low carb baked pita chips or baked corn tortillas.

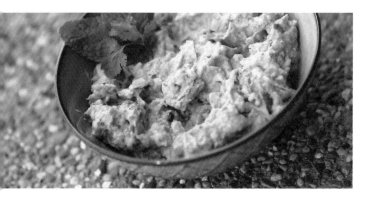

CHICKEN WINGS WITH SAUERKRAUT: "SO EASY A CAVEMAN CAN DO IT"

1 package of frozen precooked boneless or traditional chicken wings *(preferably low-fat)*

homemade probiotic boost cilantro mint dip *(Page 47)*

1 cup sauerkraut, *rinsed and drained*

Bake the chicken wings at 375 degrees for 30-45 minutes till cooked well. Follow instructions to make the cilantro mint dip on page 47.

Serve with cilantro mint dip and a side of sauerkraut. Easy does it!

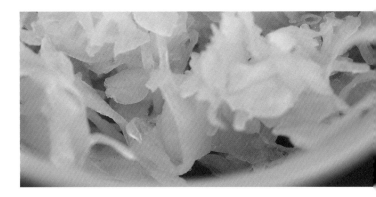

TEMPEH HERB SALAD: VEGAN RECIPE

Tempeh is an Indonesian food item. It is typically available at local ethnic grocery stores in the frozen food section. It may have black spots and white material between the soy beans which is Rhizopus Oligosporus or Rhizopus Oryzae (*the fermenting fungi*). I recommend cooking the packaged tempeh well before using it in your recipes. (**www.tofurky.com**)

12 oz. package tempeh, *frozen*

1/3 cup red onion, *chopped*

1/3 cup green pepper, *diced*

1/3 cup green peas, *boiled*

1/3 teaspoon garlic paste

1/4 teaspoon fresh ginger paste

1/2 cup baby carrots, *steamed until soft*

1/4 cup celery, *chopped*

1/4 teaspoon oregano powder

1/4 teaspoon dried parsley

1/4 cup fresh cilantro leaves

2-3 teaspoons soy sauce

1 cup low-fat mayonnaise

1/2 teaspoon dijon mustard

1 teaspoon lemon juice

1. Defrost and steam cook the tempeh for 20-25 minutes.

2. Grate or break tempeh into small pieces. Mix it with mustard, mayonnaise, soy sauce, garlic paste, ginger paste and oregano powder.

3. Let it marinate for about 2 hours in a refrigerator for the flavors to sink in.

4. Add the remaining ingredients and mix well. May add some lemon juice and sea salt, to taste.

5. Garnish with dry rosemary leaves. Mix well, serve as a salad or on a sandwich.

Caution: This recipe is for those foodies who like to experiment. Not everyone may like the taste of tempeh.

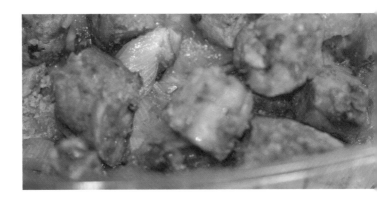

REFERENCES

1. The role of probiotics and prebiotics in inducing gut immunity Angélica T. Vieira et al Frontiers in Immunology | Mucosal Immunity December 2013 | Volume 4 | Article 445 | Immunopharmacology Group, Department of Biochemistry and Immunology, Institute of Biological Sciences, Federal University of Minas Gerais, Belo Horizonte, Brazil, Department of Microbiology.

2. A Gastroenterologist's Guide to Probiotics Matthew A Ciorba. A Gastroenterologist's Guide to Probiotics. Vol. 10, No. 9, Department of Medicine, Division of Gastroenterology, Washington University, St Louis School of Medicine, St Louis, Missouri.

3. To review the potential risks associated with probiotics please visit the department of health and human services website. http://www.ncbi.nlm.nih.gov/books/NBK56091/pdf/TOC.pdf

4. Novel probiotic Enterococcus faecium IS-27526 supplementation increased total salivary IgA level and bodyweight of preschool children: A pilot study. Surono el Al. Anaerobe. 2011 Dec;17(6):496-500. doi: 10.1016/j.anaerobe.2011.06.003. Epub 2011 Jul 5.

5. Safety of Probiotics to Reduce Risk and Prevent or Treat Disease. Molecular Biology, Genetics and Biotechnology Volume 17, Issue 6, December 2011, Pages 496–500 AHRQ Publication No. 11-E007 April 2011 http://www.ncbi.nlm.nih.gov/books/NBK56091/pdf/TOC.pdf

6. Prophylactic use of a probiotic in the prevention of colic, regurgitation and functional constipation: a randomized clinical trial. Indrio F et al JAMA Pediatr. 2014 Mar 1;168(3):228-33. doi: 10.1001/jama pediatrics.2013.4367.

7. Lactobacillus acidophilus NCFM affects colonic mucosal opioid receptor expression in patients with functional abdominal pain — a randomised clinical study. Ringel-Kulka T et al Aliment Pharmacol Ther. 2014 May 22. doi: 10.1111/apt. 12800.

8. A Lactobacillus casei Shirota probiotic drink reduces antibiotic-associated diarrhea in patients with spinal cord injuries: a randomised controlled trial. Br J Nutr. 2014 Feb;111(4):672-8. doi: 10.1017/S0007114513002973. Epub 2013 Sep 18. Wong S et al

9. Clinical trial: a multistrain probiotic preparation significantly reduces symptoms of irritable bowel syndrome in a double-blind placebo-controlled study. Pharmacol Ther. 2009 Jan;29(1):97-103. doi: 10.1111/j.1365-2036.2008.03848.x. Epub 2008 Sep 9. Williams EA et al

10. www.FoodnavigatorUSA.com

11. www.consumerlab.com

INDEX

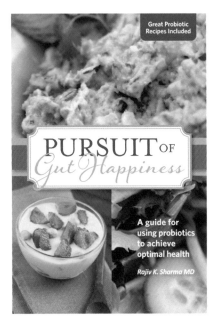

CPSIA information can be obtained at www.ICGtesting.com
Printed in the USA
LVIW01n2329050415
433364LV00002B/2